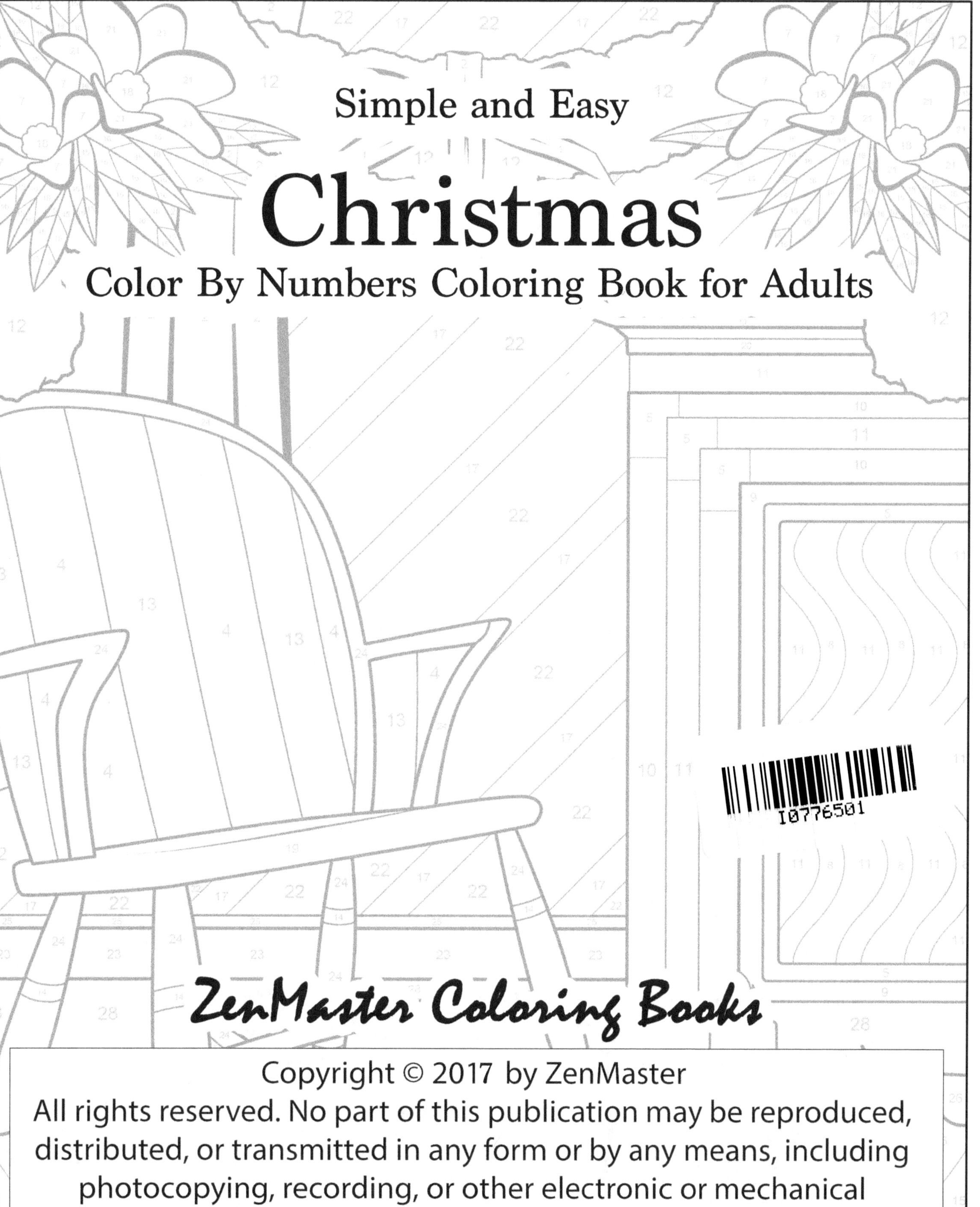

Simple and Easy

Christmas

Color By Numbers Coloring Book for Adults

ZenMaster Coloring Books

Helpful Tips for Coloring

~ Sometimes the colors appear differently on paper than what you would expect. Use the color test page to play with your colors beforehand.

~ If you are using colored pencils make sure to keep them sharp. This helps when coloring smaller areas or details on the page. Fine point sharpies also work great for smaller areas.

~ Speaking of sharpies, make sure you put a scrap piece of paper behind the page you are coloring to keep the markers from bleeding to the next page.

~ When using crayons or pencils start out light. You can always go back and darken later.

~ There are so many tools for coloring: markers, sharpies, crayons, pencils, pastels, and the list goes on. Experiment with what works best for you and your designs. Though it's not necessary, using higher quality coloring utensils makes a difference.

~ If you come to a design that seems overwhelming just pick a place to start and go from there. Once you begin your creativity will quickly take over!! If you get discouraged just take a break and come back to the page later.

~ Remember to practice. Like anything else, the more you do it the better you'll get. It'll become more and more relaxing each time.

~ DON'T FOLLOW THE RULES! It's up to you how you color your designs. Just let your creativity take the lead and HAVE FUN!

COLOR TEST PAGE

COLOR TEST PAGE

1. Baby Pink
2. Rose Pink
3. Poinsett Red
4. Dark Red
5. Magenta Haze
6. Plum
7. Blue Violet
8. Snowflake
9. Tiffany Blue
10. Teal
11. Blue
12. Christmas Green
13. Green
14. Apple Green
15. Pine Green
16. Dark Green
17. Canary Yellow
18. Lemon Yellow
19. Naples Yellow
20. Dark Gold
21. Amber
22. Chestnut
23. Cocoa Brown
24. Wood Brown
25. Silver
26. Dim Grey
27. Charcoal
28. Dark Grey

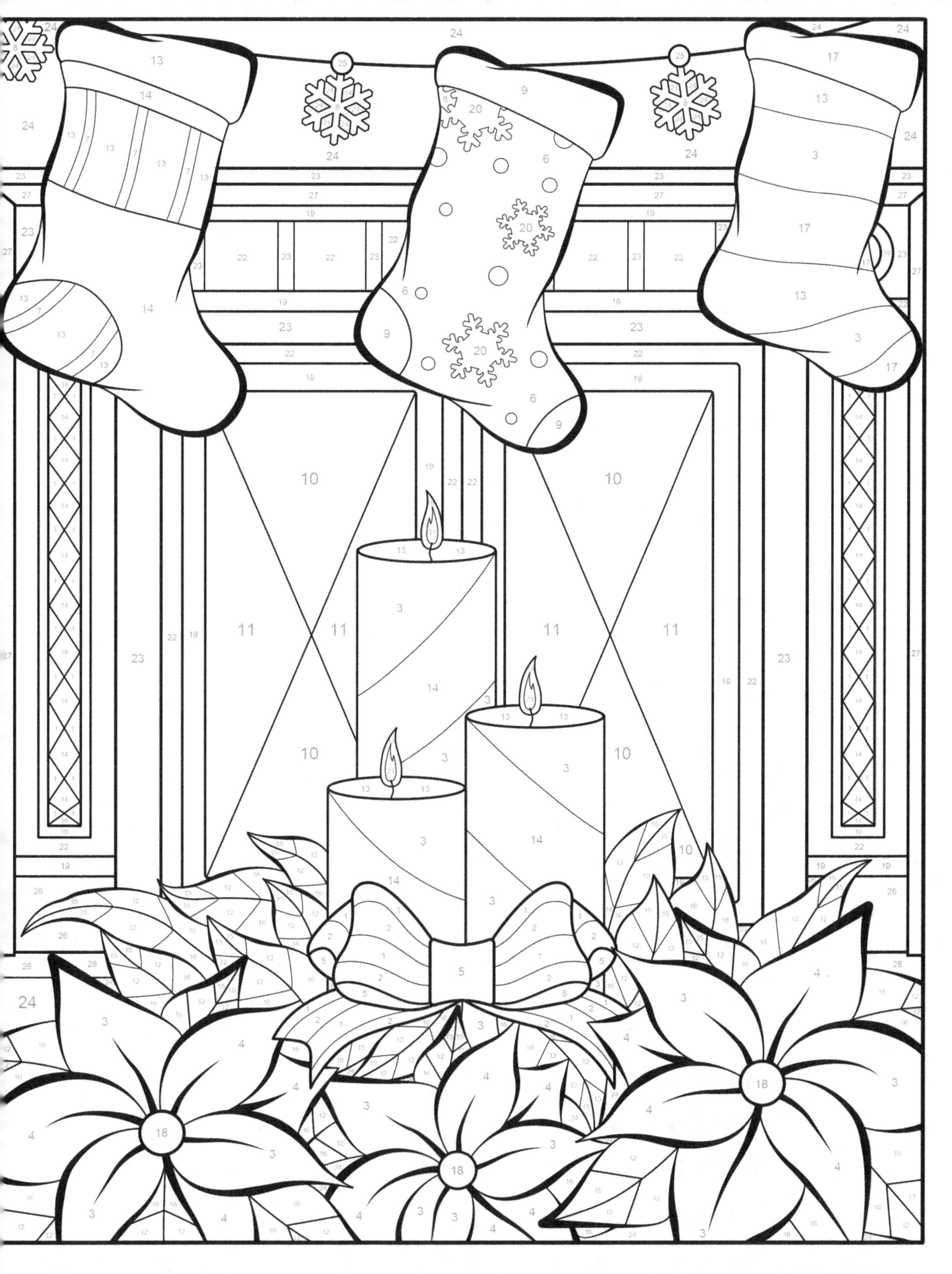

1. Baby Pink
2. Rose Pink
3. Poinsett Red
4. Dark Red
5. Magenta Haze
6. Plum
7. Blue Violet
8. Snowflake
9. Tiffany Blue
10. Teal
11. Blue
12. Christmas Green
13. Green
14. Apple Green
15. Pine Green
16. Dark Green
17. Canary Yellow
18. Lemon Yellow
19. Naples Yellow
20. Dark Gold
21. Amber
22. Chestnut
23. Cocoa Brown
24. Wood Brown
25. Silver
26. Dim Grey
27. Charcoal
28. Dark Grey

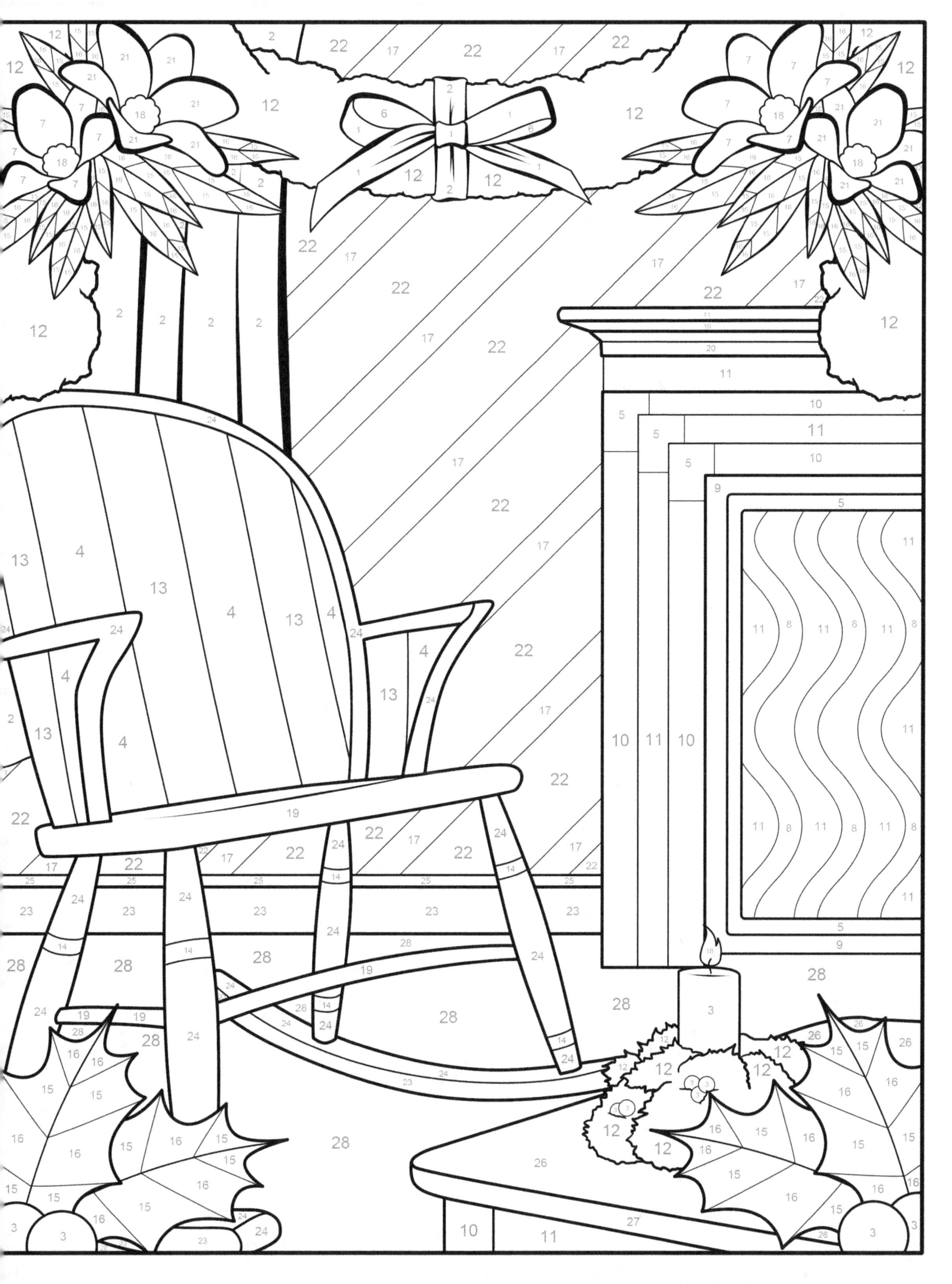

1. Baby Pink
2. Rose Pink
3. Poinsett Red
4. Dark Red
5. Magenta Haze
6. Plum
7. Blue Violet
8. Snowflake
9. Tiffany Blue
10. Teal
11. Blue
12. Christmas Green
13. Green
14. Apple Green
15. Pine Green
16. Dark Green
17. Canary Yellow
18. Lemon Yellow
19. Naples Yellow
20. Dark Gold
21. Amber
22. Chestnut
23. Cocoa Brown
24. Wood Brown
25. Silver
26. Dim Grey
27. Charcoal
28. Dark Grey

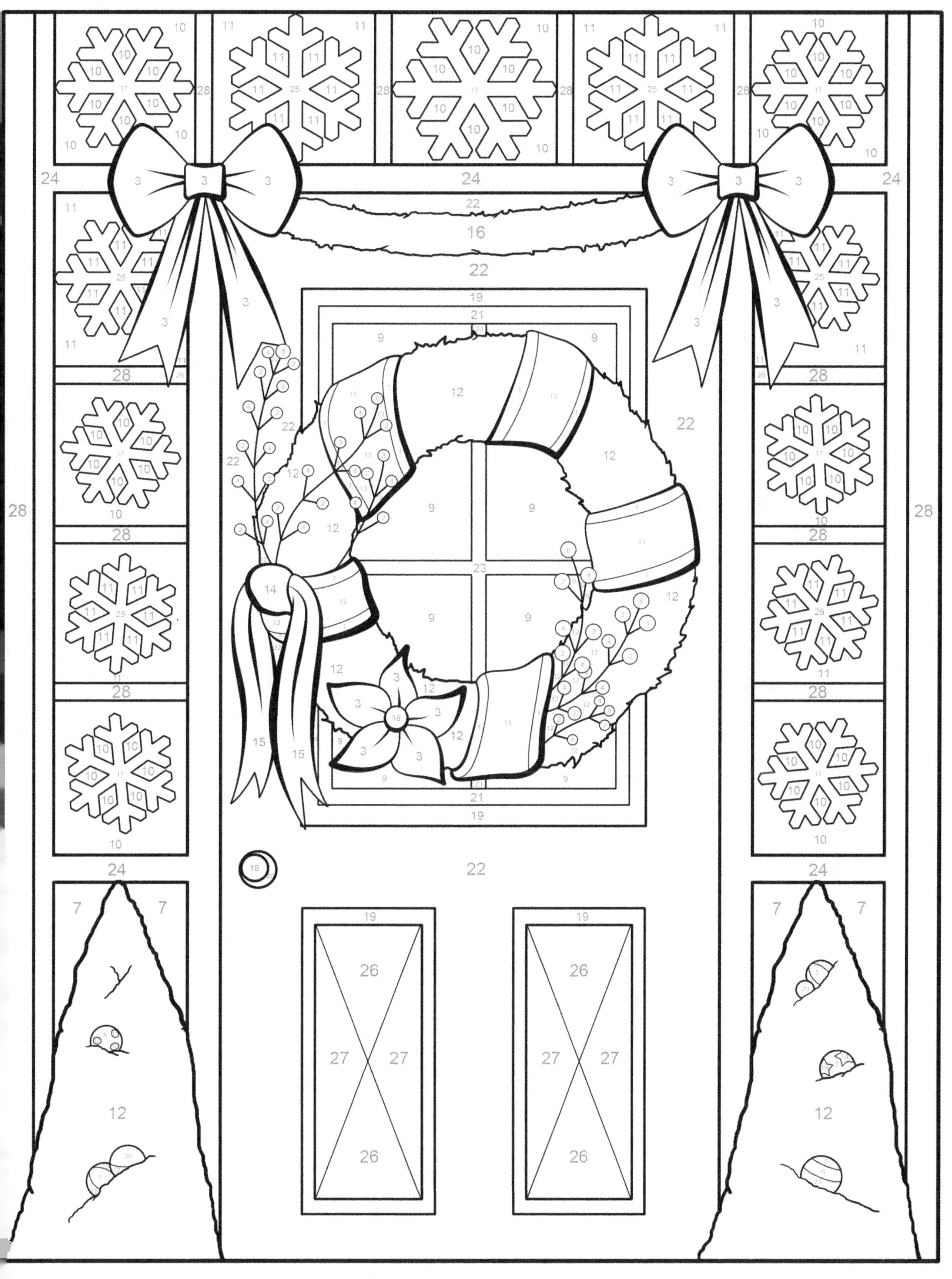

1. Baby Pink
2. Rose Pink
3. Poinsett Red
4. Dark Red
5. Magenta Haze
6. Plum
7. Blue Violet
8. Snowflake
9. Tiffany Blue
10. Teal
11. Blue
12. Christmas Green
13. Green
14. Apple Green
15. Pine Green
16. Dark Green
17. Canary Yellow
18. Lemon Yellow
19. Naples Yellow
20. Dark Gold
21. Amber
22. Chestnut
23. Cocoa Brown
24. Wood Brown
25. Silver
26. Dim Grey
27. Charcoal
28. Dark Grey

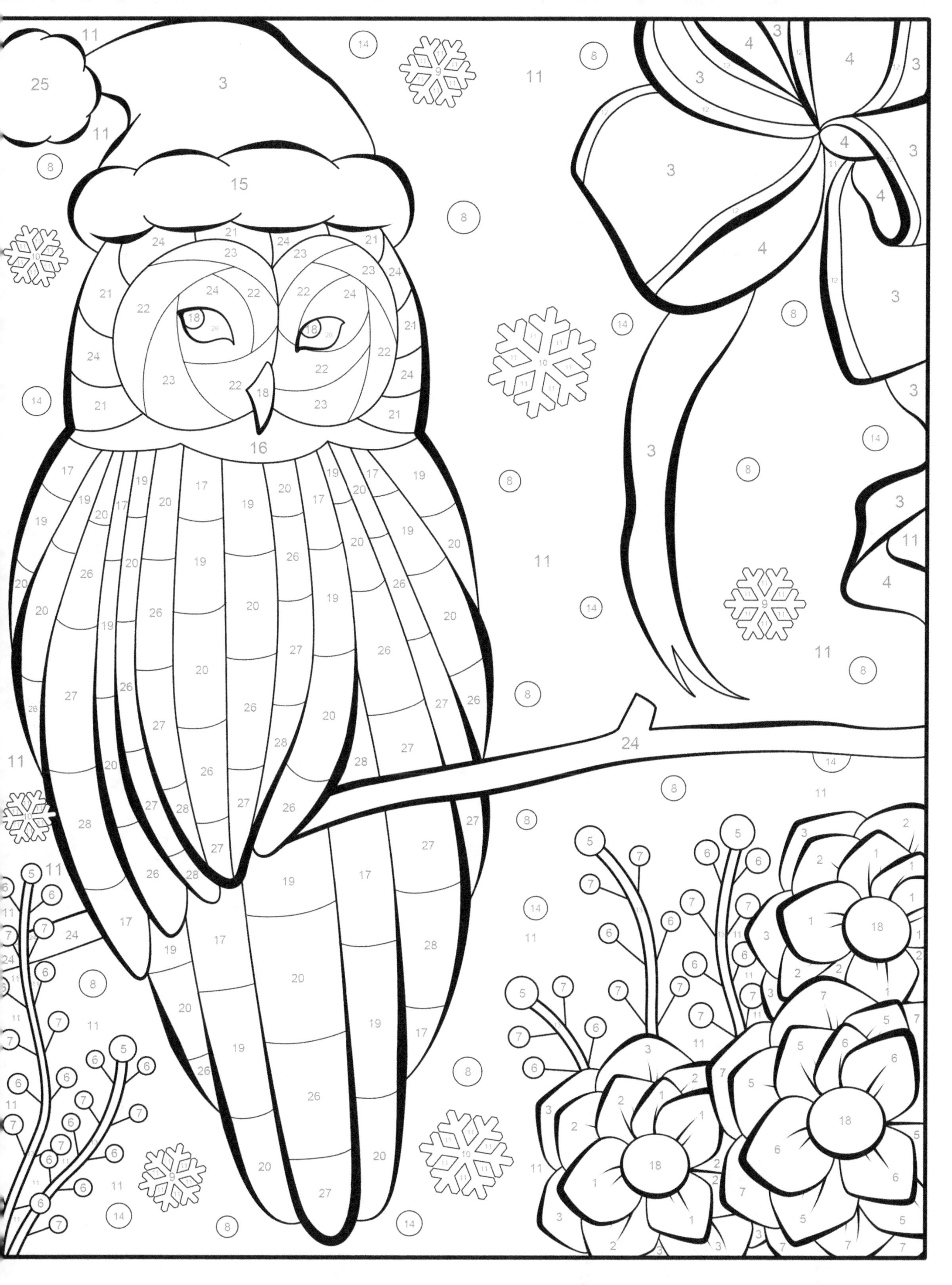

1. Baby Pink
2. Rose Pink
3. Poinsett Red
4. Dark Red
5. Magenta Haze
6. Plum
7. Blue Violet
8. Snowflake
9. Tiffany Blue
10. Teal
11. Blue
12. Christmas Green
13. Green
14. Apple Green
15. Pine Green
16. Dark Green
17. Canary Yellow
18. Lemon Yellow
19. Naples Yellow
20. Dark Gold
21. Amber
22. Chestnut
23. Cocoa Brown
24. Wood Brown
25. Silver
26. Dim Grey
27. Charcoal
28. Dark Grey

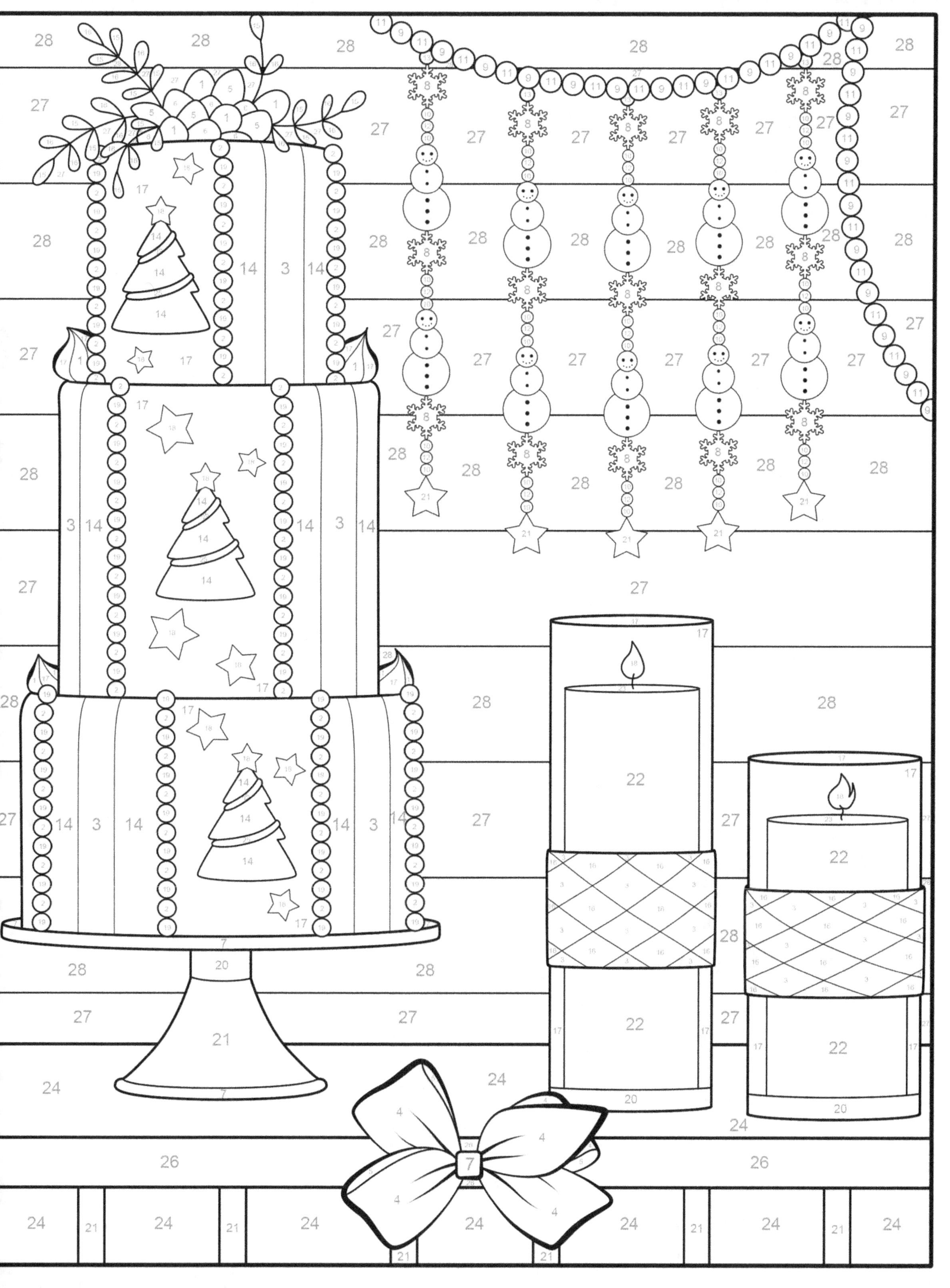

1. Baby Pink
2. Rose Pink
3. Poinsett Red
4. Dark Red
5. Magenta Haze
6. Plum
7. Blue Violet
8. Snowflake
9. Tiffany Blue
10. Teal
11. Blue
12. Christmas Green
13. Green
14. Apple Green
15. Pine Green
16. Dark Green
17. Canary Yellow
18. Lemon Yellow
19. Naples Yellow
20. Dark Gold
21. Amber
22. Chestnut
23. Cocoa Brown
24. Wood Brown
25. Silver
26. Dim Grey
27. Charcoal
28. Dark Grey

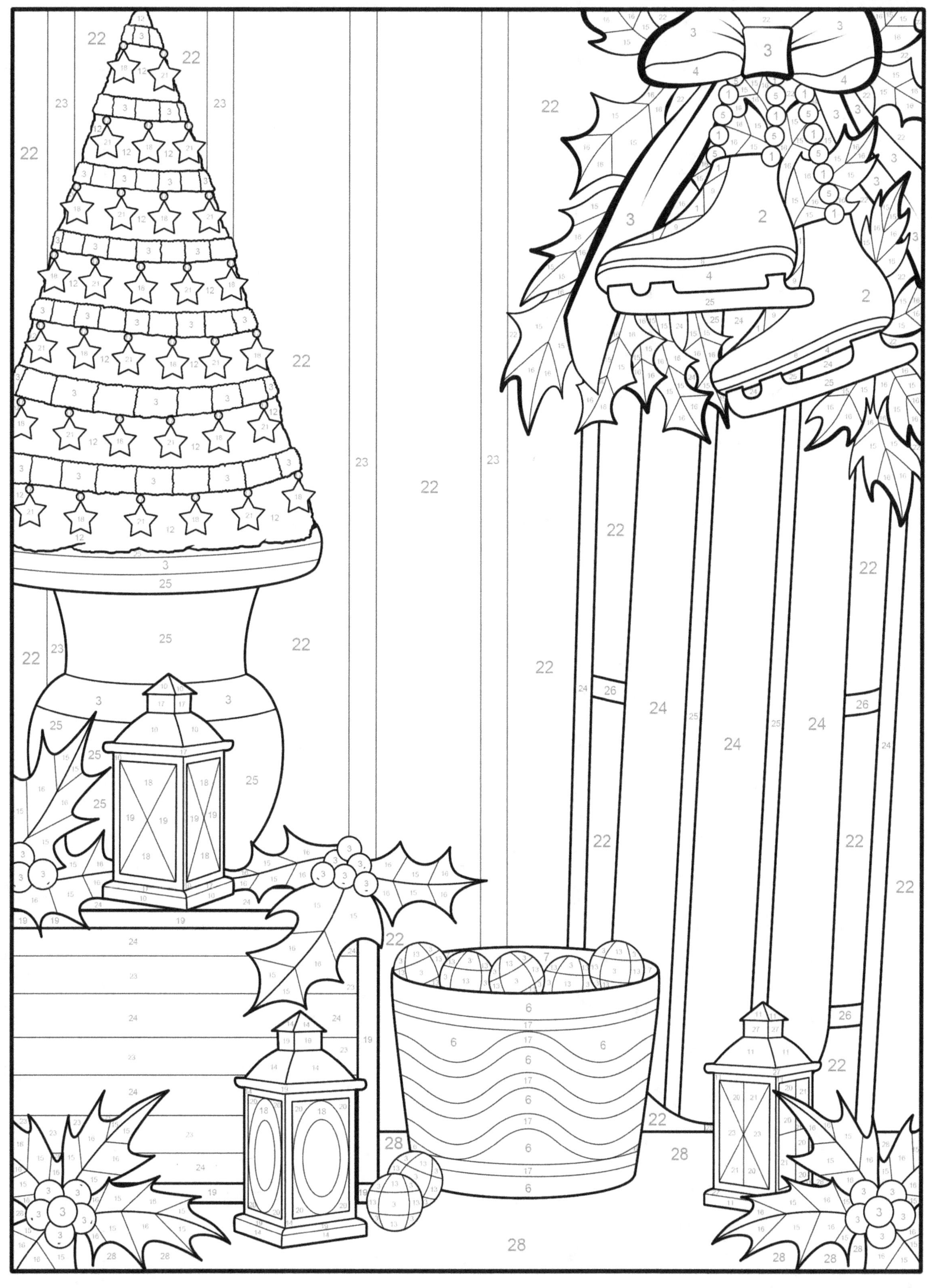

1. Baby Pink
2. Rose Pink
3. Poinsett Red
4. Dark Red
5. Magenta Haze
6. Plum
7. Blue Violet
8. Snowflake
9. Tiffany Blue
10. Teal
11. Blue
12. Christmas Green
13. Green
14. Apple Green
15. Pine Green
16. Dark Green
17. Canary Yellow
18. Lemon Yellow
19. Naples Yellow
20. Dark Gold
21. Amber
22. Chestnut
23. Cocoa Brown
24. Wood Brown
25. Silver
26. Dim Grey
27. Charcoal
28. Dark Grey

1. Baby Pink
2. Rose Pink
3. Poinsett Red
4. Dark Red
5. Magenta Haze
6. Plum
7. Blue Violet
8. Snowflake
9. Tiffany Blue
10. Teal
11. Blue
12. Christmas Green
13. Green
14. Apple Green
15. Pine Green
16. Dark Green
17. Canary Yellow
18. Lemon Yellow
19. Naples Yellow
20. Dark Gold
21. Amber
22. Chestnut
23. Cocoa Brown
24. Wood Brown
25. Silver
26. Dim Grey
27. Charcoal
28. Dark Grey

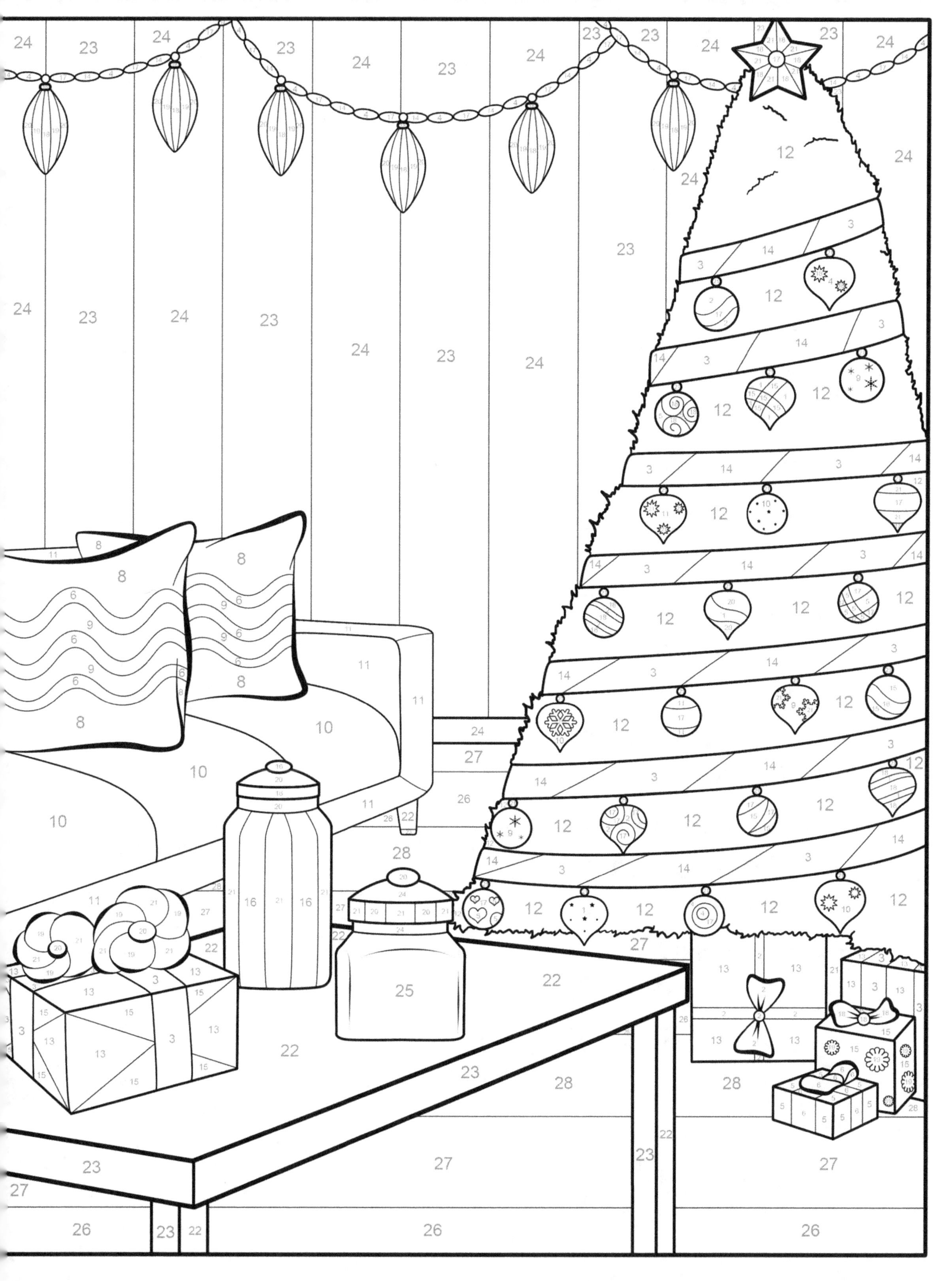

1. Baby Pink
2. Rose Pink
3. Poinsett Red
4. Dark Red
5. Magenta Haze
6. Plum
7. Blue Violet
8. Snowflake
9. Tiffany Blue
10. Teal
11. Blue
12. Christmas Green
13. Green
14. Apple Green
15. Pine Green
16. Dark Green
17. Canary Yellow
18. Lemon Yellow
19. Naples Yellow
20. Dark Gold
21. Amber
22. Chestnut
23. Cocoa Brown
24. Wood Brown
25. Silver
26. Dim Grey
27. Charcoal
28. Dark Grey

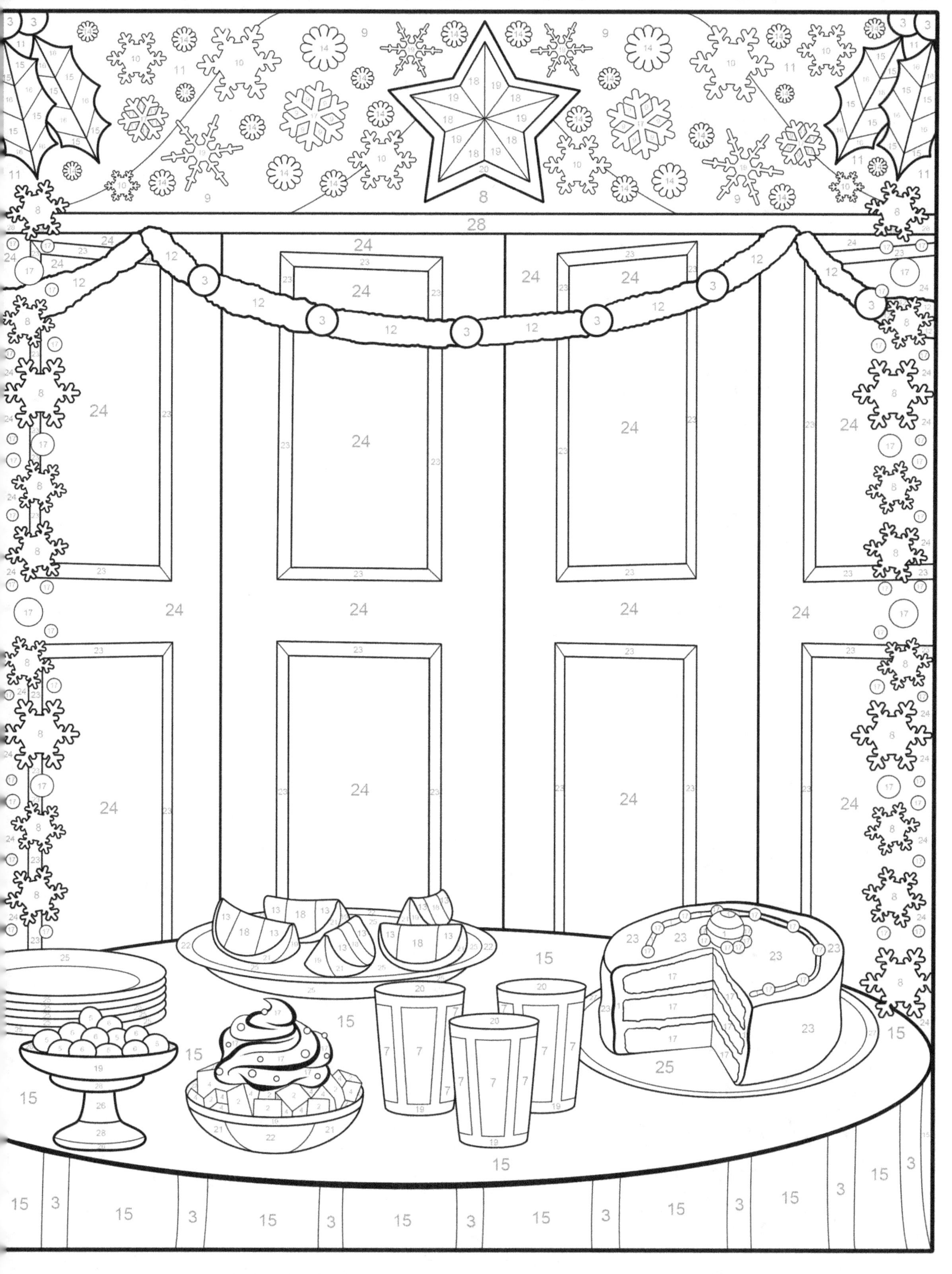

1. Baby Pink
2. Rose Pink
3. Poinsett Red
4. Dark Red
5. Magenta Haze
6. Plum
7. Blue Violet
8. Snowflake
9. Tiffany Blue
10. Teal
11. Blue
12. Christmas Green
13. Green
14. Apple Green
15. Pine Green
16. Dark Green
17. Canary Yellow
18. Lemon Yellow
19. Naples Yellow
20. Dark Gold
21. Amber
22. Chestnut
23. Cocoa Brown
24. Wood Brown
25. Silver
26. Dim Grey
27. Charcoal
28. Dark Grey

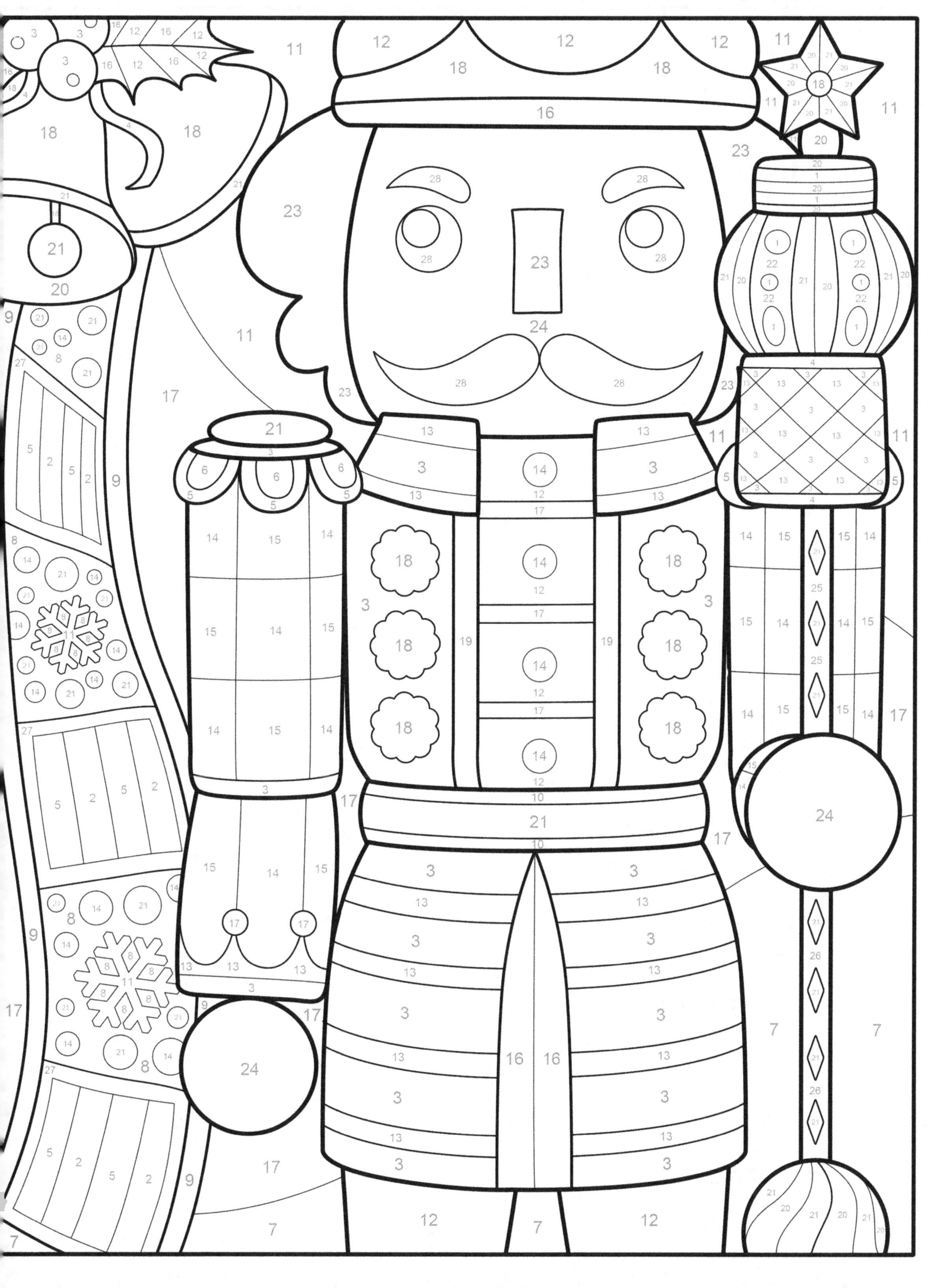

1. Baby Pink
2. Rose Pink
3. Poinsett Red
4. Dark Red
5. Magenta Haze
6. Plum
7. Blue Violet
8. Snowflake
9. Tiffany Blue
10. Teal
11. Blue
12. Christmas Green
13. Green
14. Apple Green
15. Pine Green
16. Dark Green
17. Canary Yellow
18. Lemon Yellow
19. Naples Yellow
20. Dark Gold
21. Amber
22. Chestnut
23. Cocoa Brown
24. Wood Brown
25. Silver
26. Dim Grey
27. Charcoal
28. Dark Grey

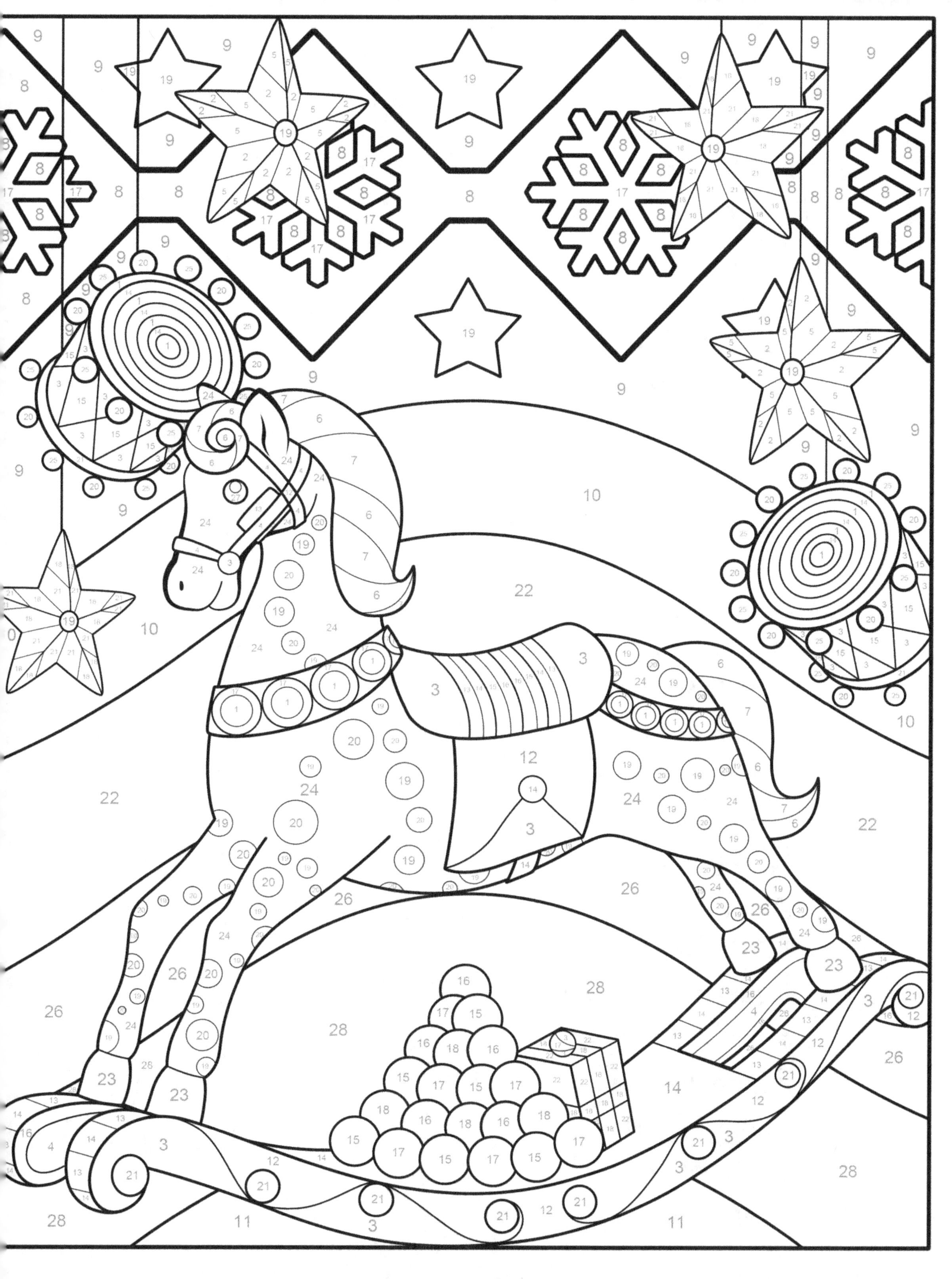

1. Baby Pink
2. Rose Pink
3. Poinsett Red
4. Dark Red
5. Magenta Haze
6. Plum
7. Blue Violet
8. Snowflake
9. Tiffany Blue
10. Teal
11. Blue
12. Christmas Green
13. Green
14. Apple Green
15. Pine Green
16. Dark Green
17. Canary Yellow
18. Lemon Yellow
19. Naples Yellow
20. Dark Gold
21. Amber
22. Chestnut
23. Cocoa Brown
24. Wood Brown
25. Silver
26. Dim Grey
27. Charcoal
28. Dark Grey

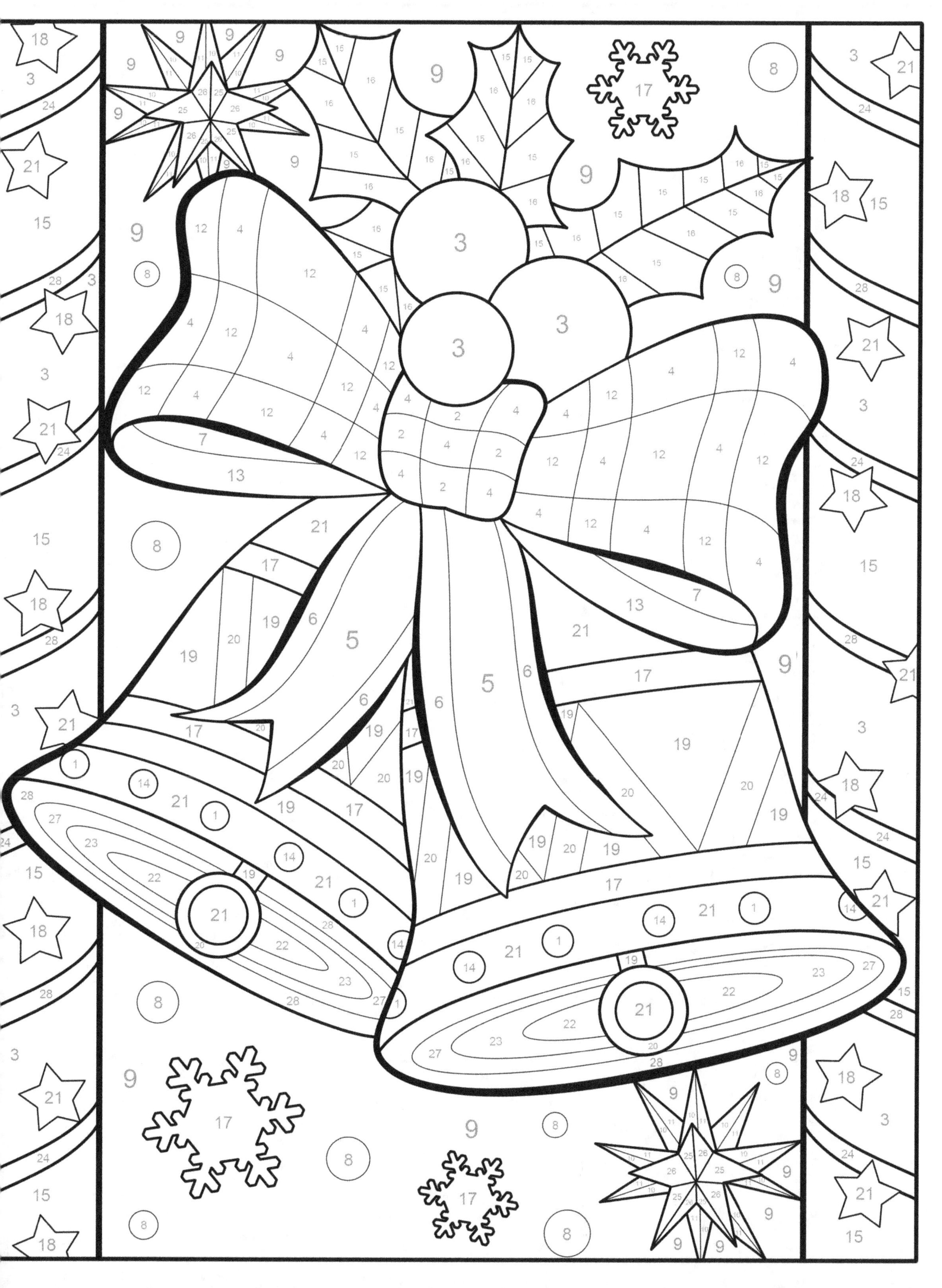

1. Baby Pink
2. Rose Pink
3. Poinsett Red
4. Dark Red
5. Magenta Haze
6. Plum
7. Blue Violet
8. Snowflake
9. Tiffany Blue
10. Teal
11. Blue
12. Christmas Green
13. Green
14. Apple Green
15. Pine Green
16. Dark Green
17. Canary Yellow
18. Lemon Yellow
19. Naples Yellow
20. Dark Gold
21. Amber
22. Chestnut
23. Cocoa Brown
24. Wood Brown
25. Silver
26. Dim Grey
27. Charcoal
28. Dark Grey

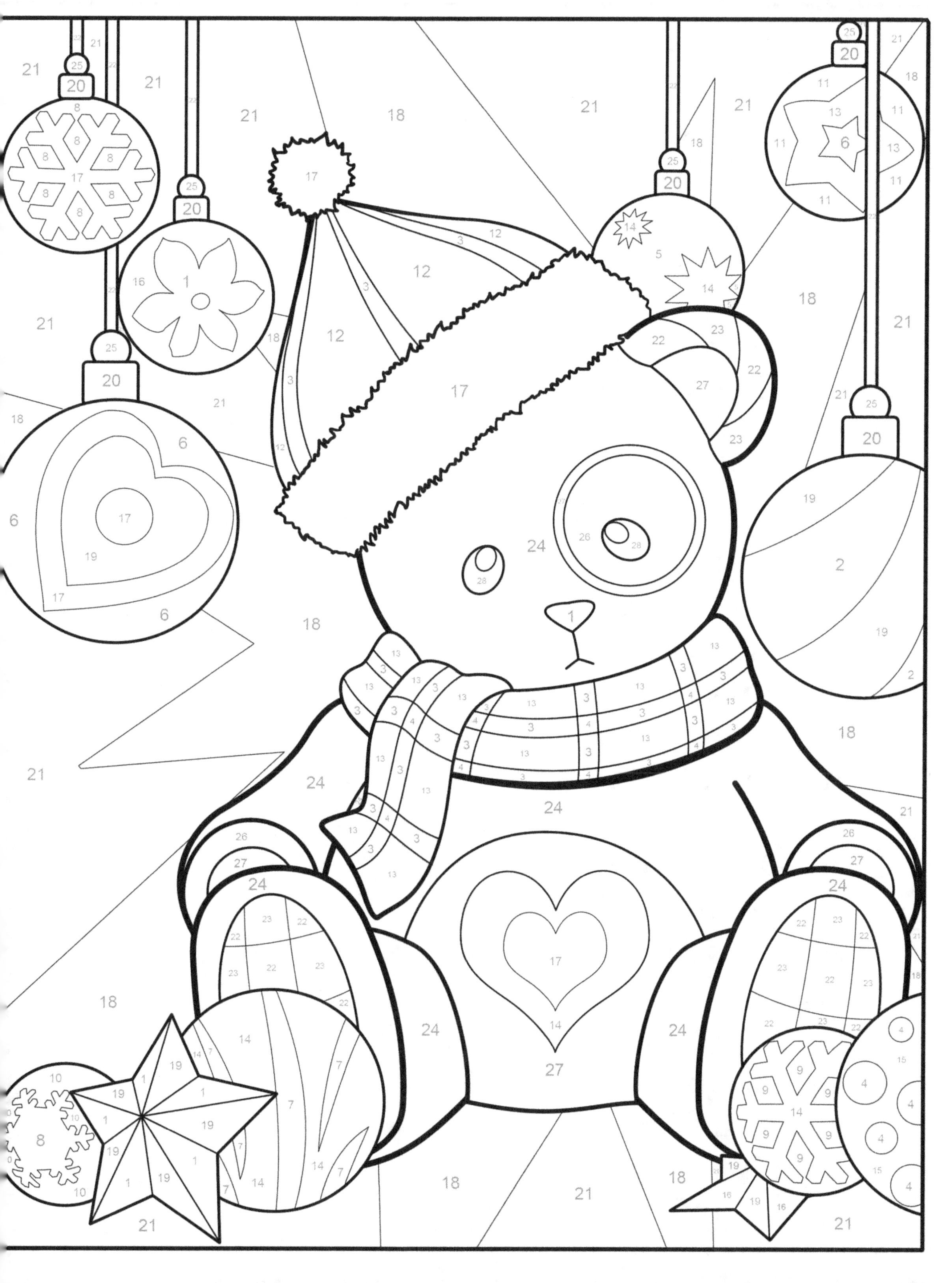

1. Baby Pink
2. Rose Pink
3. Poinsett Red
4. Dark Red
5. Magenta Haze
6. Plum
7. Blue Violet
8. Snowflake
9. Tiffany Blue
10. Teal
11. Blue
12. Christmas Green
13. Green
14. Apple Green
15. Pine Green
16. Dark Green
17. Canary Yellow
18. Lemon Yellow
19. Naples Yellow
20. Dark Gold
21. Amber
22. Chestnut
23. Cocoa Brown
24. Wood Brown
25. Silver
26. Dim Grey
27. Charcoal
28. Dark Grey

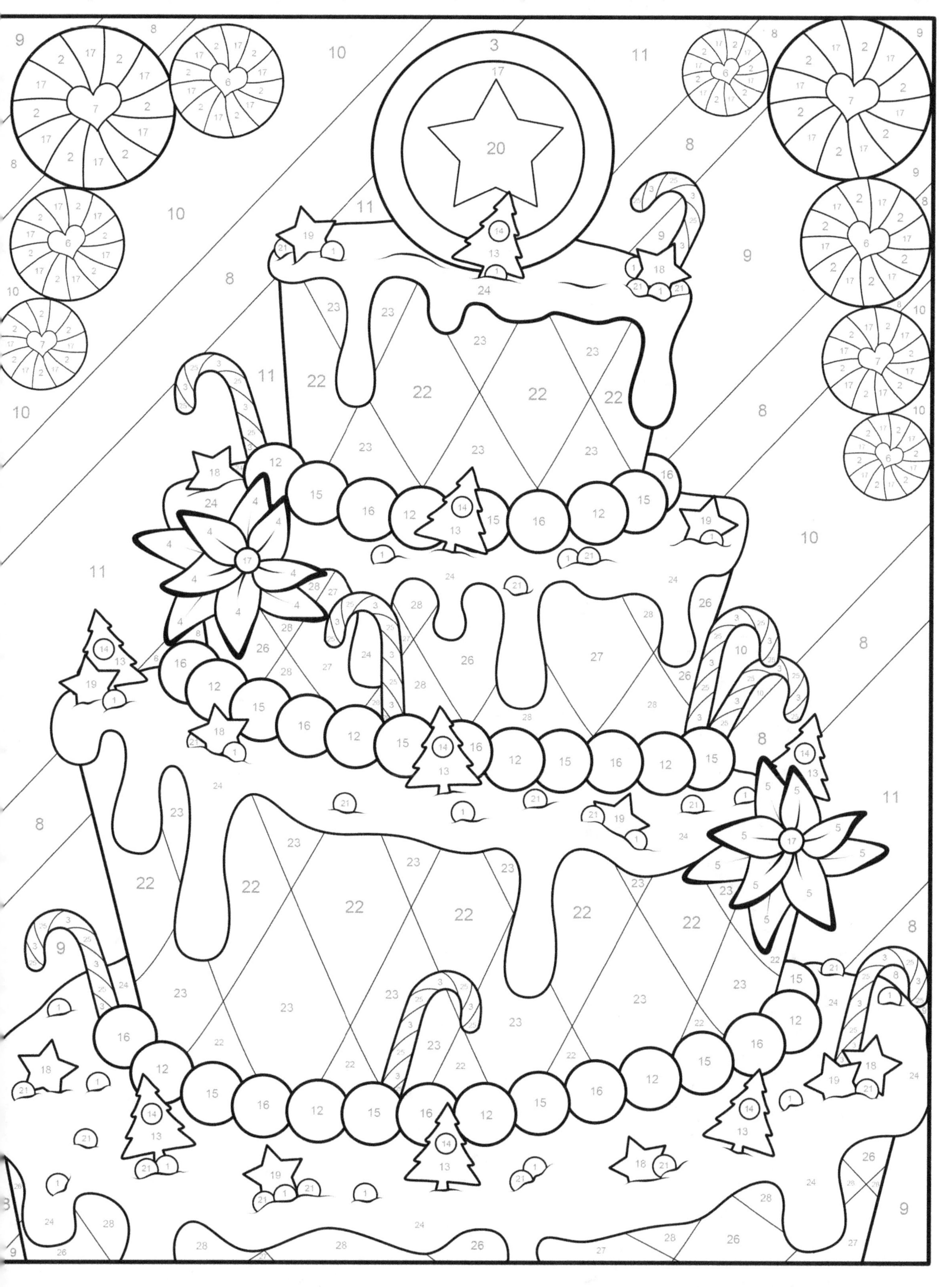

1. Baby Pink
2. Rose Pink
3. Poinsett Red
4. Dark Red
5. Magenta Haze
6. Plum
7. Blue Violet
8. Snowflake
9. Tiffany Blue
10. Teal
11. Blue
12. Christmas Green
13. Green
14. Apple Green
15. Pine Green
16. Dark Green
17. Canary Yellow
18. Lemon Yellow
19. Naples Yellow
20. Dark Gold
21. Amber
22. Chestnut
23. Cocoa Brown
24. Wood Brown
25. Silver
26. Dim Grey
27. Charcoal
28. Dark Grey

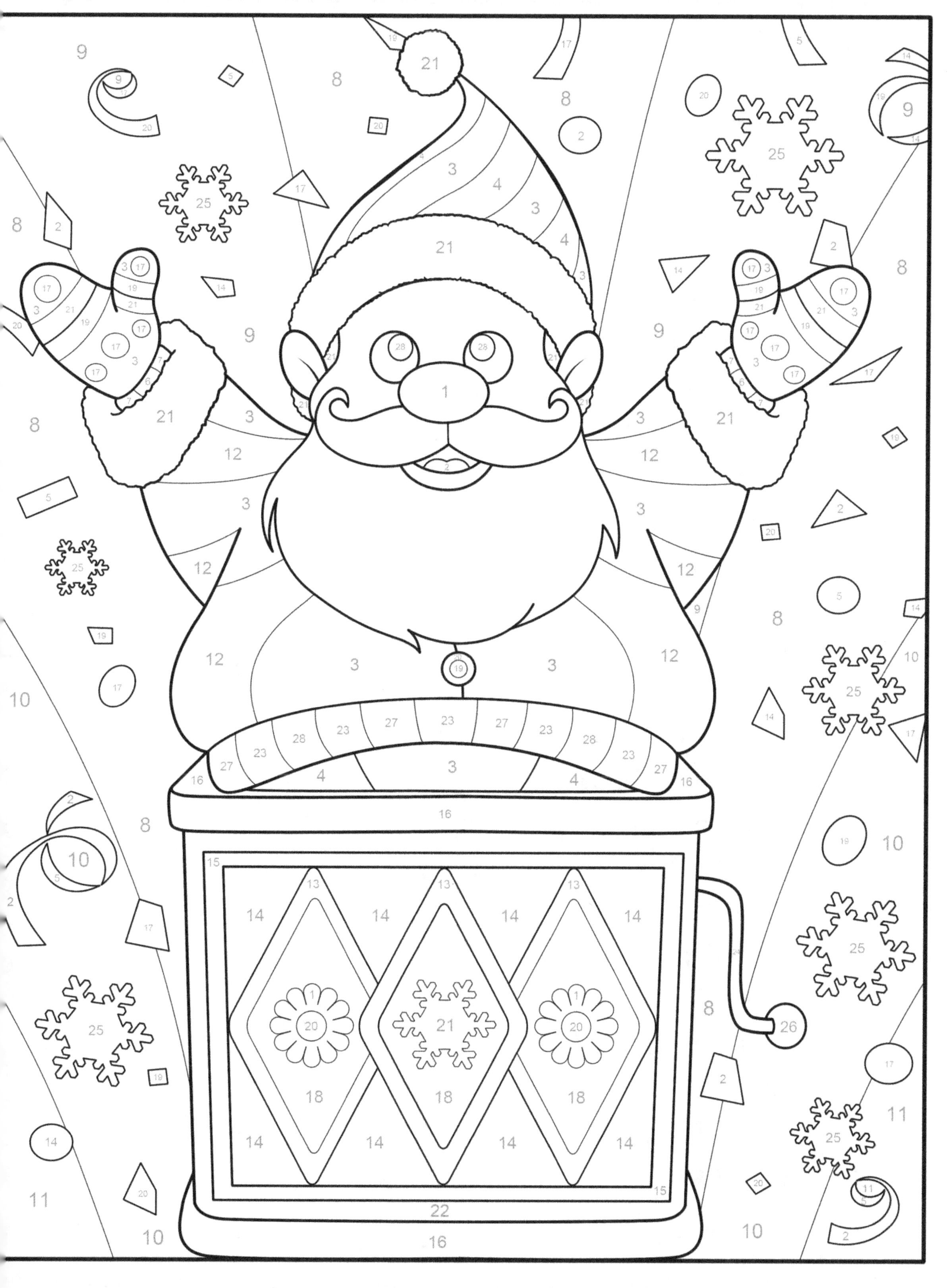

1. Baby Pink
2. Rose Pink
3. Poinsett Red
4. Dark Red
5. Magenta Haze
6. Plum
7. Blue Violet
8. Snowflake
9. Tiffany Blue
10. Teal
11. Blue
12. Christmas Green
13. Green
14. Apple Green
15. Pine Green
16. Dark Green
17. Canary Yellow
18. Lemon Yellow
19. Naples Yellow
20. Dark Gold
21. Amber
22. Chestnut
23. Cocoa Brown
24. Wood Brown
25. Silver
26. Dim Grey
27. Charcoal
28. Dark Grey

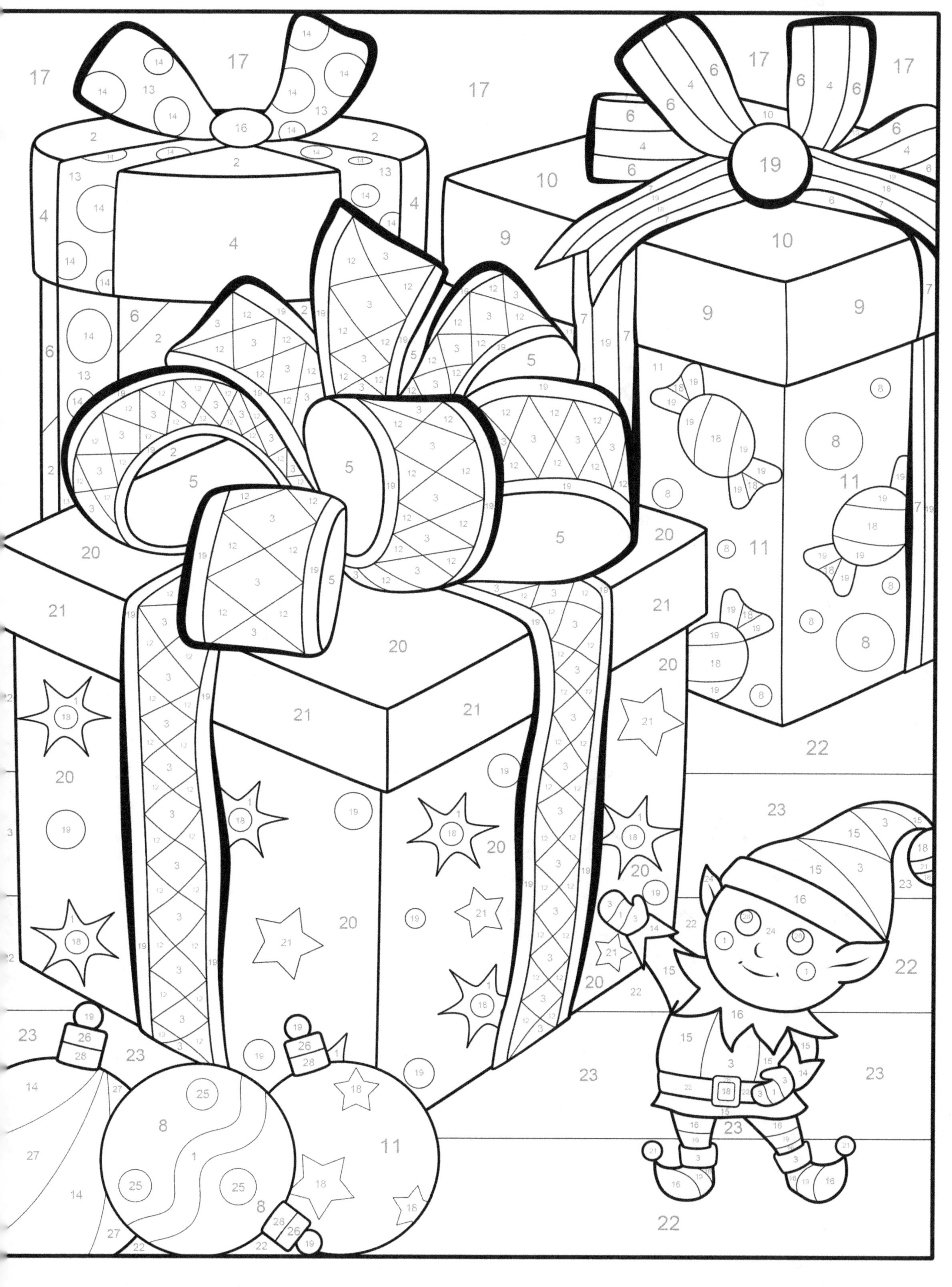

1. Baby Pink
2. Rose Pink
3. Poinsett Red
4. Dark Red
5. Magenta Haze
6. Plum
7. Blue Violet
8. Snowflake
9. Tiffany Blue
10. Teal
11. Blue
12. Christmas Green
13. Green
14. Apple Green
15. Pine Green
16. Dark Green
17. Canary Yellow
18. Lemon Yellow
19. Naples Yellow
20. Dark Gold
21. Amber
22. Chestnut
23. Cocoa Brown
24. Wood Brown
25. Silver
26. Dim Grey
27. Charcoal
28. Dark Grey

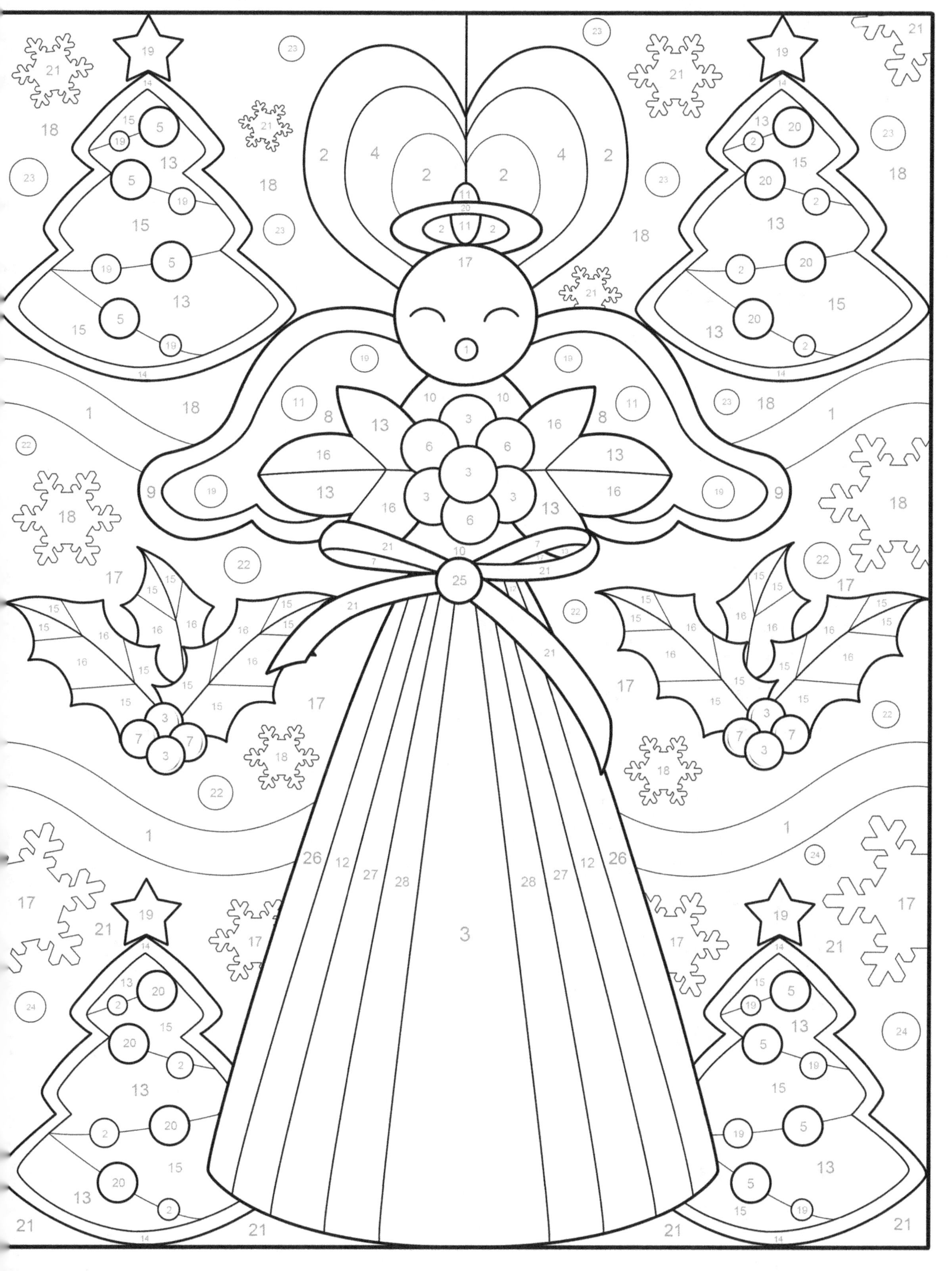

1. Baby Pink
2. Rose Pink
3. Poinsett Red
4. Dark Red
5. Magenta Haze
6. Plum
7. Blue Violet
8. Snowflake
9. Tiffany Blue
10. Teal
11. Blue
12. Christmas Green
13. Green
14. Apple Green
15. Pine Green
16. Dark Green
17. Canary Yellow
18. Lemon Yellow
19. Naples Yellow
20. Dark Gold
21. Amber
22. Chestnut
23. Cocoa Brown
24. Wood Brown
25. Silver
26. Dim Grey
27. Charcoal
28. Dark Grey

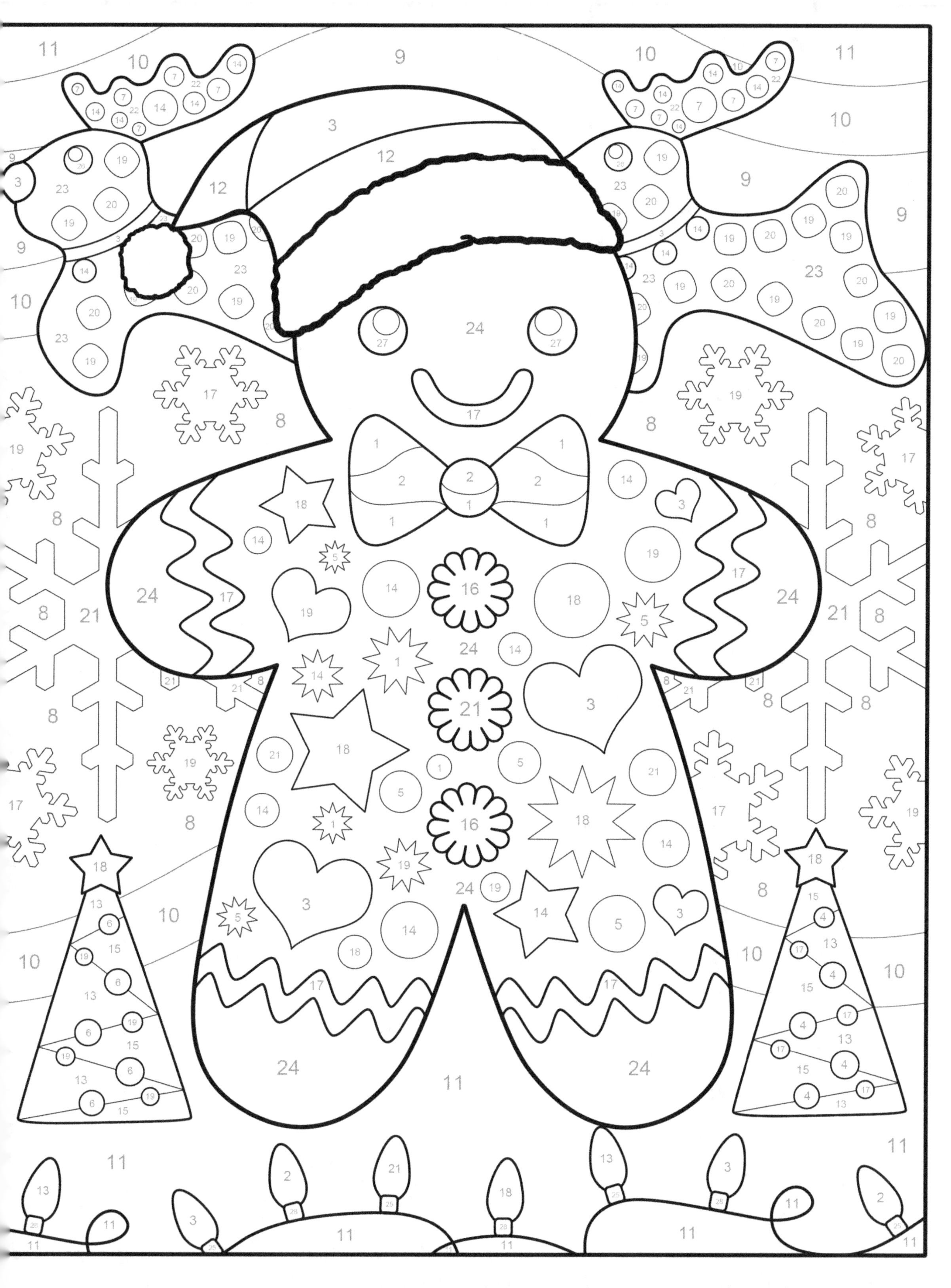

1. Baby Pink
2. Rose Pink
3. Poinsett Red
4. Dark Red
5. Magenta Haze
6. Plum
7. Blue Violet
8. Snowflake
9. Tiffany Blue
10. Teal
11. Blue
12. Christmas Green
13. Green
14. Apple Green
15. Pine Green
16. Dark Green
17. Canary Yellow
18. Lemon Yellow
19. Naples Yellow
20. Dark Gold
21. Amber
22. Chestnut
23. Cocoa Brown
24. Wood Brown
25. Silver
26. Dim Grey
27. Charcoal
28. Dark Grey

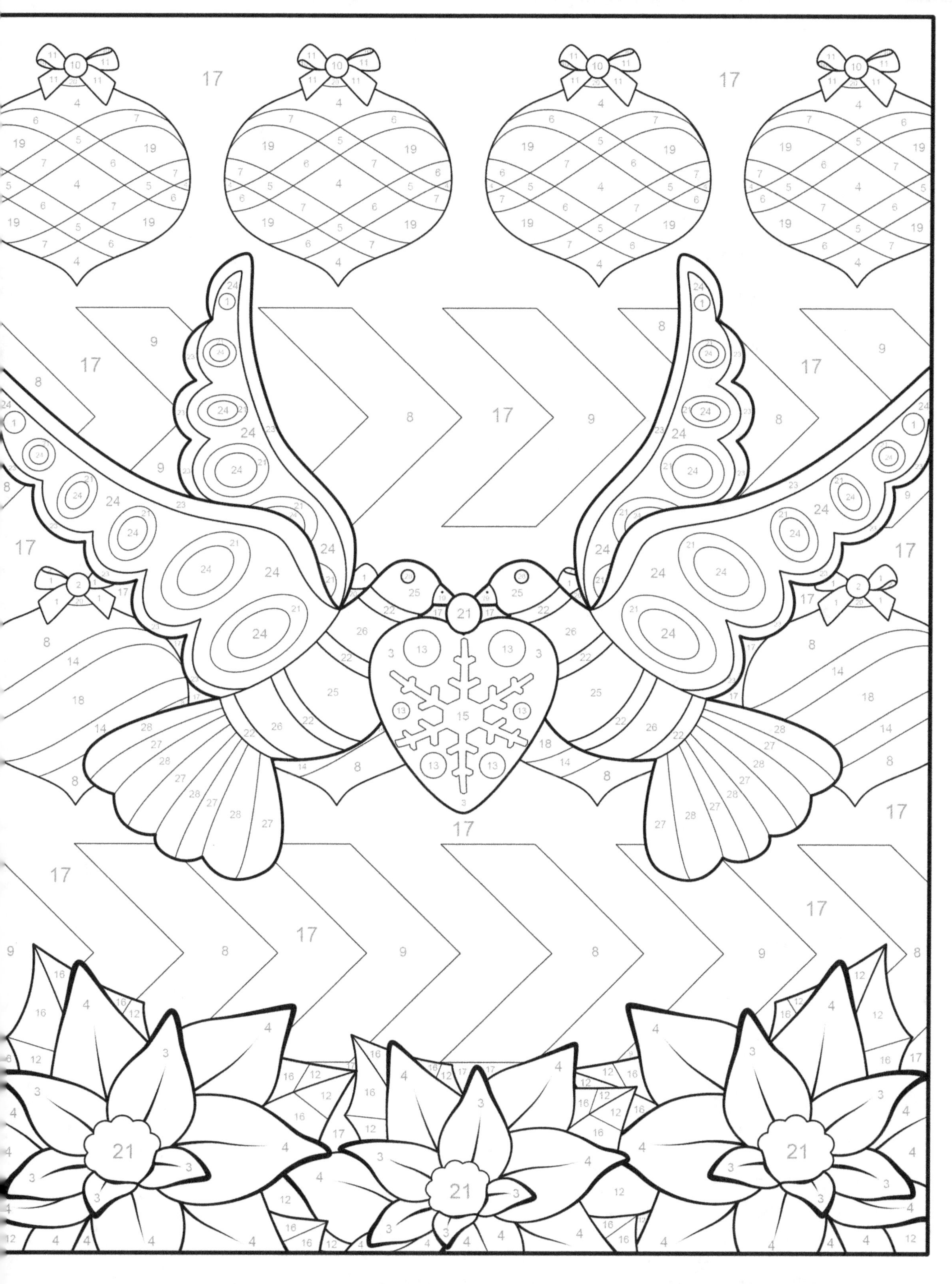

1. Baby Pink
2. Rose Pink
3. Poinsett Red
4. Dark Red
5. Magenta Haze
6. Plum
7. Blue Violet
8. Snowflake
9. Tiffany Blue
10. Teal
11. Blue
12. Christmas Green
13. Green
14. Apple Green
15. Pine Green
16. Dark Green
17. Canary Yellow
18. Lemon Yellow
19. Naples Yellow
20. Dark Gold
21. Amber
22. Chestnut
23. Cocoa Brown
24. Wood Brown
25. Silver
26. Dim Grey
27. Charcoal
28. Dark Grey

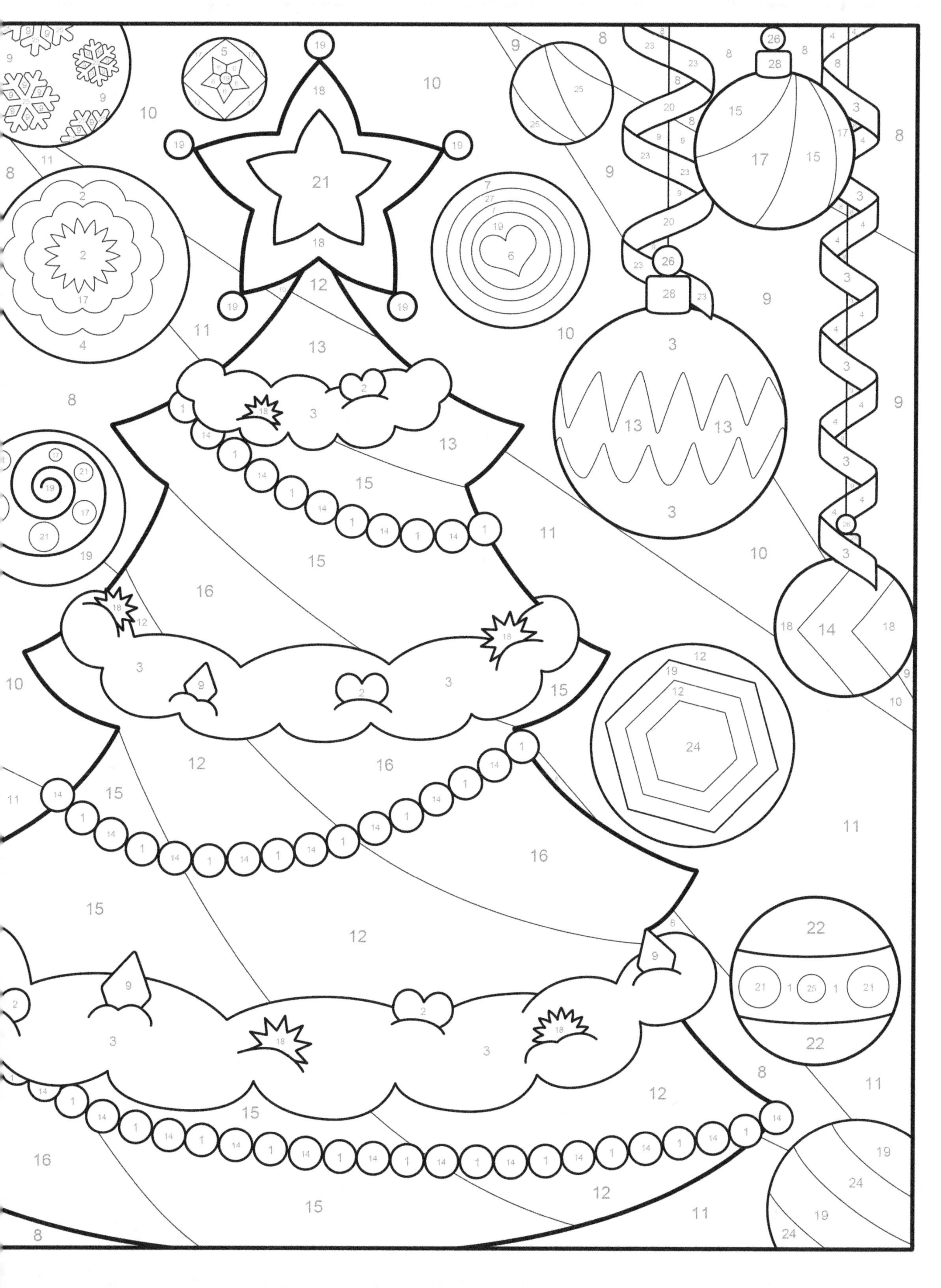

Thank you for supporting
ZenMaster Coloring Books

Your support means the world to us,
and we're thrilled to have you embark on this
creative journey with us.

Our small company strives to make a
BIG difference by helping those
who may be less fortunate.

This is why we proudly hire struggling
artists from around the world!

Our goal is to provide financial support to artists and
their families by enabling them to pursue their passions
and share their hard work and limitless talent with you!

Help support our hard working artists
by leaving a positive review on Amazon!

And follow us on Facebook for updates and
FREE COLORING PAGES!
https://www.facebook.com/zenmastercoloringbooks/

Check out more of our books at:
amazon.com/author/zenmastercoloringbooks

Free Bonus Page!
from:

Large Print Adult Coloring Book of
Kittens and Cats

https://www.amazon.com/dp/1983684775

Also available in color by numbers!!

https://www.amazon.com/dp/1983687626

And 5x8" Travel Size

https://www.amazon.com/dp/1727552121

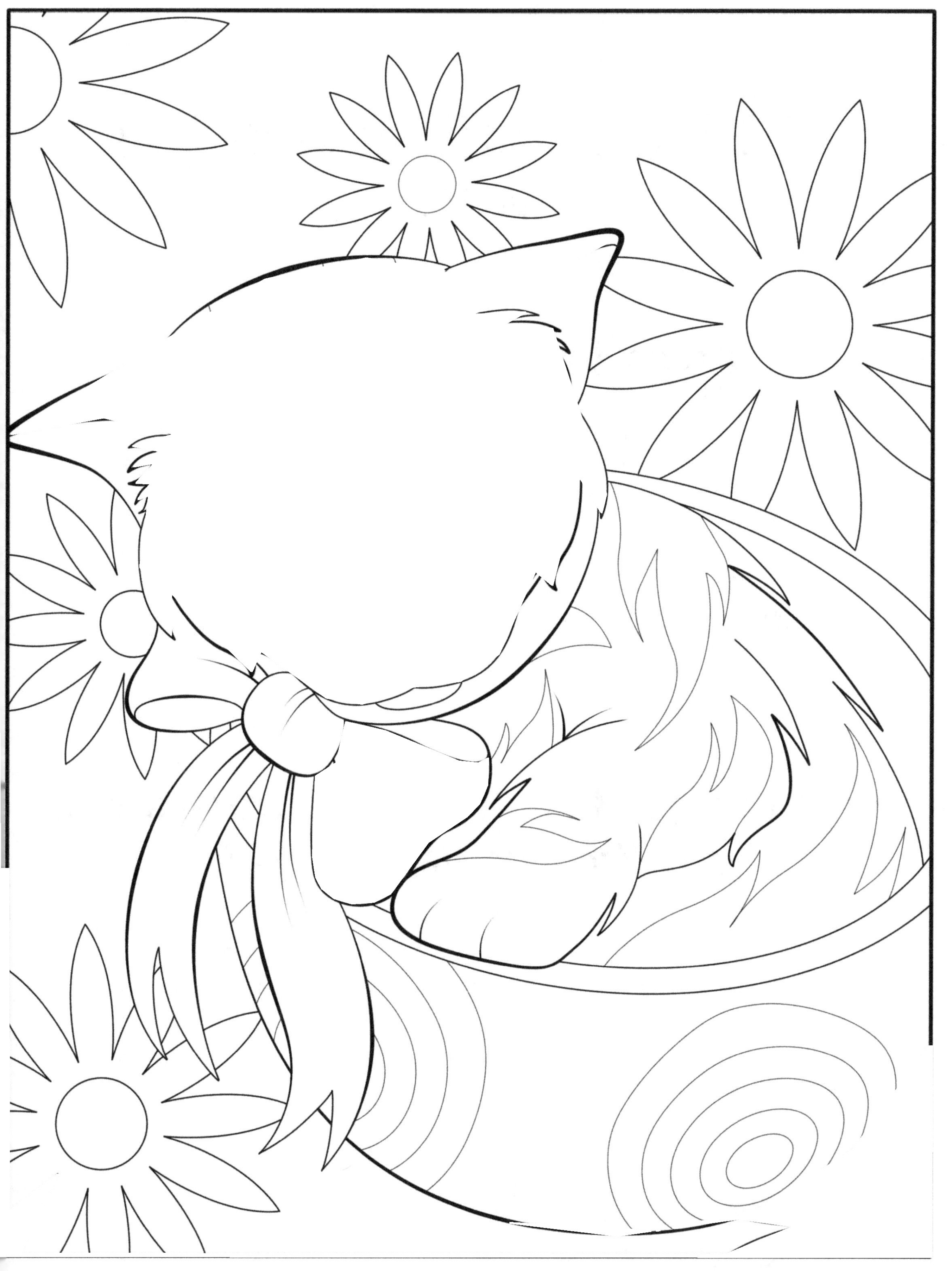

Free Bonus Page!
from:

Large Print Simple and Easy
Mandalas

https://www.amazon.com/dp/198151290x

Also available in color by numbers!!
https://amzn.com/dp/198207616x

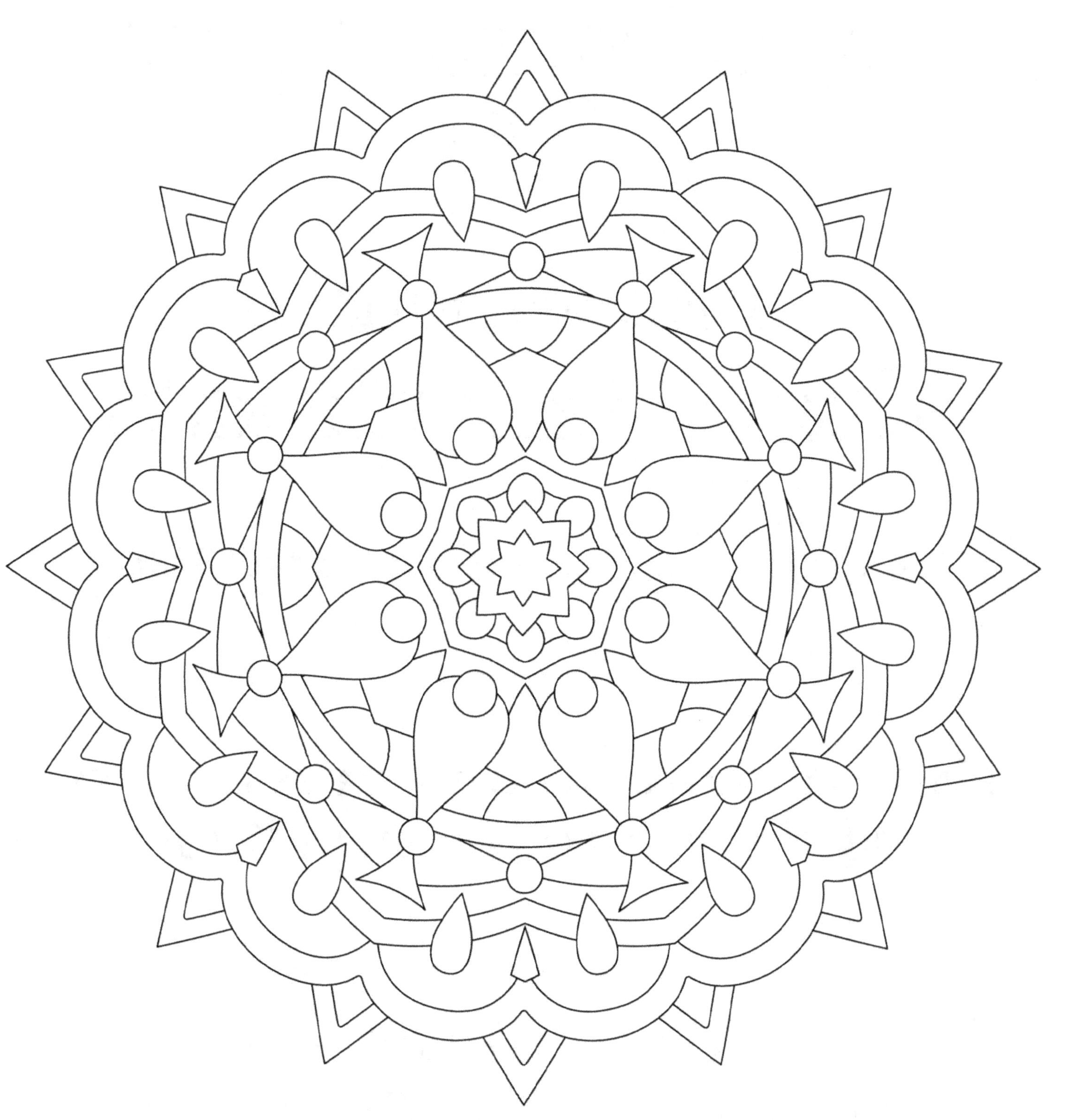

Free Bonus Page!
from:

Adult Coloring Book of
Sweets and Treats

https://www.amazon.com/dp/1795668881

Also available in color by numbers!!

https://www.amazon.com/dp/1795670983

And 5x8" Travel Size

https://www.amazon.com/dp/1796511447

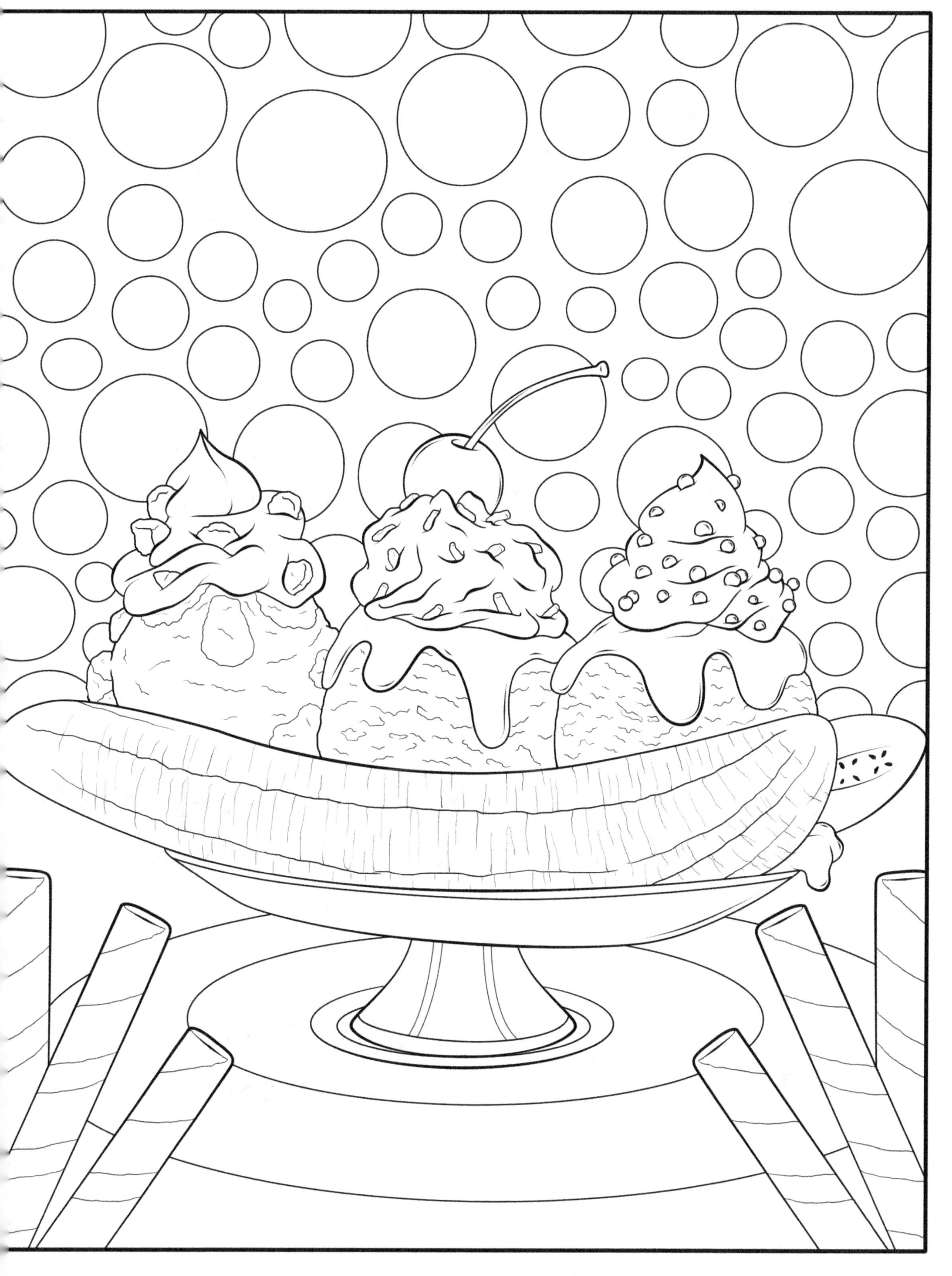

Free Bonus Page!
from:

Winter Wonderland
Large Print Coloring Book for Adults

https://www.amazon.com/dp/1979068704

Also available in color by numbers!!
https://www.amazon.com/dp/1979269661

And 5x8" Travel Size
https://www.amazon.com/dp/1726194647

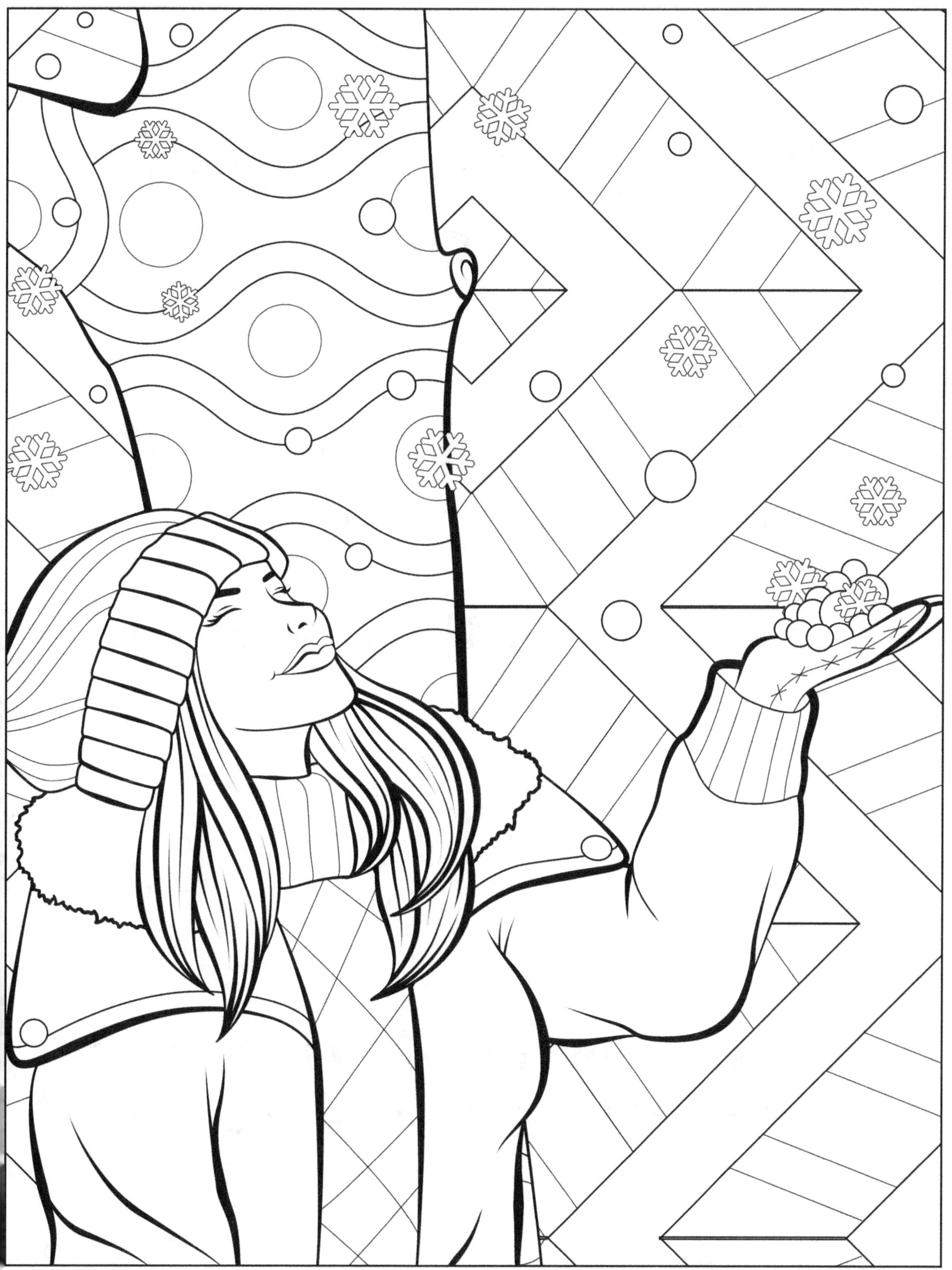

Free Bonus Page!
from:

Zen Coloring Notebook

https://www.amazon.com/dp/1535457015

Available in 9 different colors!

Also available in 5x8" journal size

https://www.amazon.com/dp/1535540591